The Split Brain

The Split Brain

An Analysis of Schizophrenia

Aurealia N. Nelson

Writers Club Press
San Jose New York Lincoln Shanghai

The Split Brain
An Analysis of Schizophrenia

All Rights Reserved © 2001 by Aurealia N. Nelson

No part of this book may be reproduced or transmitted in any form or by any means, graphic, electronic, or mechanical, including photocopying, recording, taping, or by any information storage retrieval system, without the permission in writing from the publisher.

Writers Club Press
an imprint of iUniverse.com, Inc.

For information address:
iUniverse.com, Inc.
5220 S 16th, Ste. 200
Lincoln, NE 68512
www.iuniverse.com

ISBN: 0-595-18314-X

Printed in the United States of America

To all those who believed in me.

An Analysis of Schizophrenia

ABSTRACT

For individuals struck with the disorder, schizophrenia is a life-shattering event which curtails careers, breaks up families, forfends any possibility of financial stability, leads to severe physiological, psychological and social impairments, and, in many cases (up to 15% of schizophrenics according to some studies) to death through suicide (APA, 1997; Carter and Flesher, 1995; Wyatt, et al., 1996). Schizophrenia's impact reaches beyond just schizophrenics and their immediate families. This is for the families and the search for meaning in the madness.

Introduction

One out of every one hundred persons suffers at some time in his or her life from either Schizophrenia or symptoms of the manic-depressive. This high incidence of a usually debilitating condition has led to excessive experimentation and research to get at the causes of the disease. However, despite the work involved and the progress made in finding factors peculiar to schizophrenics, there is little agreement on the causes of Schizophrenia and little knowledge of the cure, if any. Thus, a person diagnosed as a schizophrenic, treated and released as being cured, has a great chance of returning to treatment or of merely resuming his suffering.

The schizophrenias are a group of psychotic disorders characterized by gross distortions of reality, withdrawal from social interaction, and disorganization and fragmentation of perception, thought and emotion (Tollefson, 1996). Schizophrenia is a comparatively rare disorder—the incidence rate is only about 0.01% and the lifetime prevalence rate across a variety of populations worldwide is typically estimated at about 1% (Larsen and Opjordsmoen, 1996; APA, 1997, p. 6). Yet, despite its relatively low incidence (when compared to other major mental and neurological disorders) schizophrenia exerts a devastating impact on its victims, their families, and society at large. In the U.S., schizophrenia accounts for 2.5% of all total direct health care expenditures (APA, 1997, p. 7). It is estimated that 80% of schizophrenics are chronically unemployed and that schizophrenics account for 10% of the totally and permanently disabled (APA, 1997, p. 7). There are strong links between homelessness and schizophrenia, with studies suggesting that upwards of one-third of all homeless adults in the U.S. suffer from the disorder (Holzman, 1996; Carter and Flesher, 1995).

This report will draw upon the literature to explore the topic of schizophrenia. It will identify the nature of schizophrenia, including its history, etiology, causes, and clinical features, as well as look at genetic, neurophysiological, and environmental factors. It will investigate its distribution in the population and associated demographic characteristics. It will also explore biological, psychological and chemical treatments currently utilized, course, diagnosis, and barriers to successful social reintegration for schizophrenics and methods used to facilitate a return to mainstream society for members of this population.

DEFINITION OF SCHIZOPHRENIA

A common misunderstanding must be clarified before discussing schizophrenia. Schizophrenia is not multiple personality disorder; a disorder with which the split-brain disease is often confused. Take the following two definitions of schizophrenia, noting that within both definitions the distinction must be made that the illness is not multiple personality disorder. Definition One: Schizophrenia is a general term for a group of psychotic illnesses characterized by disturbed thinking, emotional reactions, and behaviors. Schizophrenia means split brain to describe how the thoughts and feelings may not relate to each other in a logical fashion. Often the disorder is described as split personality but this has led to it being confused with multiple personality disorder, a quite distinct condition (Hunt, 1996: 1). Definition Two: Schizophrenia is the term for a group of mental disorders marked by a variety of symptoms. Literally, the term means split brain, but contrary to a common misconception, schizophrenia does not imply a split personality, in the sense of someone acting like two different people. Not until the 20th Century was schizophrenia distinguished from other forms of psychosis (Encarta, 1997: 1).

History of Schizophrenia

Ever since schizophrenia was first identified, scientists have theorized about the cause of the illness. Emil Kraepelin was the first to differentiate the condition of Schizophrenia from other psychiatric conditions. He adopted the name dementis praecox and described the essential conditions of Schizophrenia. Kraepelin believed that the origins of schizophrenia were either a degeneration of the brain or a metabolic disorder causing the body to poison the brain. He also believed the condition to be irreversible, ending in a state of complete and permanent dementia.

Eugen Bleuler coined the term schizophrenia and formed a bridge between Kraepelin and Freud. The word Schizophrenia signifies a split, not in the personality, but between the various psychological functions. Bleuler did not entirely discount the notion of a biological basis, but he emphasized the thinking of the schizophrenic. He was the first to describe the disordered thinking of the schizophrenic, pointing out the impairment of the association of ideas. He believed most of the schizophrenic's symptoms were the result of this impairment of ideas, which he called autistic or dereistic.

Adlof Meyer, like modern scientists, saw the disease as both physical and mental. The physiological and psychological disorders resulted in progressive imbalances. The schizophrenic did not adapt to these imbalances, and this pattern of maladaptation became habitual resulting in disorganizations of thought and behavior.

Freud's influence on all of psychology can also be seen on ideas about schizophrenia. Freudian interpretation thinks of regressive schizophrenic behavior as a retreat to less mature levels of the ego. It interprets the restitutive symptoms as attempts to replace the existing world that the patient has retreated from with such phenomena as hallucinations, delusions, fantasies of world reconstruction, and peculiarities of language.

Carl Jung's interpretation of Schizophrenia is in accord with his theory of the collective unconscious and archetypes. All men have some contact with the collective unconscious as represented in dreams and universal symbols. Modern men have an overlay of personality or persons that is individual. In some persons, the collective unconscious becomes too powerful, and the atavistic tendencies of the unconscious are not brought into adjustment with modern life. The patient's past life and the archetypes that present themselves result in the particular symptoms of each case. Jung's idea of the psychic objectivity of the universal psyche is not unique, but it is uncommon in explanations of Schizophrenia. He connects Schizophrenia with the underlying drive toward self-realization. It is not all individuals who experience those drives, for there are vast portions of humanity who are unconscious and have no problems with that state. However, if an individual is of a "higher" type but for some reason has remained too long in a primitive state, he states:

> Their nature does not in the long run tolerate persistence in what is for them an unnatural stupor. As a result of their narrow conscious outlook and their cramped existence they save energy; bit by bit it

accumulates in the unconscious and finally explodes
in the form of a more or less acute neurosis.

Harry Stack Sullivan saw Schizophrenia as the result of poor interpersonal relations, especially relations between parents and children. These early relations can cause anxiety and lack of self-esteem. This results in a distortion of the patient's way of living and gets disapproval of this way of living. In other words, he or she lacks "consensual validation." The lack of consensual validation causes a schizophrenic panic.

Silvano Artisti shares this dynamic interpretation of Schizophrenia. However, Aristi formulates the mechanisms by which the patient expresses his conflicts and way of life. An example of this occurs in the area of cognition. Arieti calls the schizophrenic way of thinking paleologic based on E. Von Domarus' principle that whereas a normal person assumes identity on the basis of an identical subject, the schizophrenic, when thinking paleologically, assumes identity on the basis of an identical verb or predicate. An example is given of a patient who thought she was the Virgin Mary because she was a virgin; therefore, she was the Virgin Mary. Being a virgin is the predicate in this case. The patient used this to escape from her own ideas of unworthiness. Arieti has an interesting way to account for the biological theories of the origins of Schizophrenia. He believes that intensely disturbing emotions may bring about the resurgence of obsolete functional and neural patterns.

Changing Stigma of Mental Illness

One of the biggest obstacles to finding a better treatment for schizophrenia, or even a cure, may be the fact that there still remains a high level of stigma in this country associated with mental illness. A lack of health insurance coverage has also been cited as one of the primary reasons why so few schizophrenia patients receive appropriate treatment. Further, the patients themselves may contribute to this situation because schizophrenia is a very difficult disease to manage and to openly confront. "Despite great advances in the medical treatment of schizophrenia during the second half of this century, we remain woefully deficient in our ability to deliver that treatment to patients in need. The stigma associated with mental illness is at the root of this failure and contributes to inadequacies of health insurance coverage for mental illness, lack of information and resources among the families of patients, and the difficulties many patients have in accepting their illnesses," (Dietz, 1998: 2).

Encouraging new attitudes are developing toward Schizophrenia and mental illness. Instead of seeing madness as a total stigma, many are looking to see what they can learn from the insane and others; drug users are experimenting with states of temporary insanity themselves. Hopefully, this will lead us to a new understanding of ourselves, for who can say he or she is not in some measure schizophrenic?

Effect on the Individual, Family, and Society

For individuals struck with the disorder, schizophrenia is a life-shattering event which curtails careers, breaks up families, forfends any possibility of financial stability, and leads to severe physiological, psychological and social impairments. In many cases (up to 15% of schizophrenics according to some studies) it leads to death through suicide (APA, 1997; Carter and Flesher, 1995; Wyatt, et al., 1996). Schizophrenia's impact reaches beyond just schizophrenics and their immediate families. In the U.S., schizophrenia accounts for 2.5% of all total direct health care expenditures (APA, 1997, p. 7). It is estimated that 80% of schizophrenics are chronically unemployed and that schizophrenics account for 10% of the totally and permanently disabled (APA, 1997, p. 7). There are strong links between homelessness and schizophrenia, with studies suggesting that upwards of one-third of all homeless adults in the U.S. suffer from the disorder (Holzman, 1996; Carter and Flesher, 1995).

Occurrence and Cost

Schizophrenia affects men and women equally. However, men begin to suffer from the onset of the disease on average about five years earlier in age than women do. Of the general population, approximately 150 out of 100,000 persons suffer from schizophrenia that makes its occurrence relatively rare (Public 4). However, schizophrenia is a serious catastrophic illness for those that are affected because of its early age of onset and the devastating effects it has on the victims and their families. Despite its rarity, the disease takes up an inordinate amount of resources. "Schizophrenia fills more hospital beds than almost any other illness, and Federal figures reflect the cost of schizophrenia to be from $30 billion to $48 billion in direct medical costs, lost productivity and Social Security pensions" (Public 4).

Theories of Causes

While experts agree on the fundamentally biological basis of schizophrenia, researchers have yet to precisely identify the specific genetic links, or to stipulate the exact role of neurotransmitters, or to fully understand and explain the biology-environment interactions producing this mental disorder. Nor is a "cure" for schizophrenia within view. The different perspectives of cause will be discussed below. In many cases, the theories overlap, and schizophrenia is thought to be caused by a variety of factors.

Cause and Etiology

The great controversy in Schizophrenia is the question: is Schizophrenia caused by environmental factors or is it caused by biological factors? Many scientists have now reached the conclusion that it is a combination of both of these factors that produces the schizophrenic.

Despite remarkable advances in psychiatric medicine over the past few decades (e.g., breakthroughs in understanding the biological basis of many mental illnesses, the serotonin hypothesis and the discovery of effective treatments for Major Depression, etc.) the etiology and treatment of what is generally regarded as the most devastating of the major mental disorders — schizophrenia — largely remains a puzzle.

A number of different theories have been proposed to explain the etiology of schizophrenia. Older, exclusively psychological or psychoanalytical models include the double-bind theory and the theory of the "schizophrenic family" (which basically postulates that parents create schizophrenic responses in their offspring as a consequence of fractured family communication patterns and disturbed family relations) (Larsen & Opjordsmoen, 1996; Holzman, 1996). More recently developed, strictly biological models of the etiology of schizophrenia include theories about excessive activity of dopaminergic neurons in the mesolimbic system, cerebral abnormalities (particularly in the frontal and temporal lobes) caused by neurodevelopmental disturbances, and genetic disturbances (Larsen and Opjordsmoen, 1996; APA, 1997).

Over the past two decades, however, what has emerged as the dominant model of schizophrenia etiology has adopted a much more eclectic approach, emphasizing the multiple roles of both biological (e.g., genetic, neurological) and environmental (e.g., family, culture, socio-economic status, etc.) factors in the etiology of this disorder. The adoption of this eclectic model is largely a pragmatic response to research findings indicating that no single factor (or group of related factor) dominates in the etiology of schizophrenia. The evidence on genetic links in schizophrenia provides an example of the equivocal nature of the research findings.

Brain Chemistry as a Cause

Brain chemistry has been studied as another possible cause, and perhaps as a clue to treating schizophrenia. It is thought that dopamine or neurotransmitters in overabundance may be the possible cause of the electric storms that seize the brain. Technology that is new, like brain scanning, has also shown that there are some structural deformities in the brain of persons with schizophrenia.

Powerful psychoactive drugs are used to treat schizophrenia most commonly, due to the fact that brain chemistry imbalance is considered the primary cause at present, "The drugs that are beneficial in controlling symptoms work on certain chemical messengers. These chemicals, such as dopamine and serotonin, enable brain cells to communicate with each other. Scientists conclude that an imbalance of neurotransmitters is probably at the root of the cause" (Hunt, 1996: 1).

Some of these factors are undoubtedly neuroanatomical and neurobiological. Studies of deficit in intellectual functioning among schizophrenics, associations between risk for schizophrenia and various neurological assaults in the prenatal environment, and the results of brain imaging studies revealing various regional structural brain abnormalities among schizophrenics all provide testimony to the neurological basis of the disease (Tien, et al., 1996; Hanes, et al., 1996; Russell, et al., 1997).

The theory that schizophrenia is brought on by excess activity of the neurotransmitter dopamine is based primarily upon information concerning the mode of action of drugs that are effective in treating schizophrenia (Davison & Neale, 1986). If the biochemical activity of a therapeutically effective drug is understood, or at least hypothesized, the process for the disorder may be guessed at too. Further indirect support for the theory of excess dopamine activity comes from the literature of amphetamine psychosis. Amphetamines can produce a state that closely resembles paranoid schizophrenia, and they can exacerbate the symptomatology of a schizophrenic (Davison & Neale, 1987). It is often argued that excess dopamine activity can be blocked by phenothiazines, given rise to the belief that this may be one of the causal factors in the etiology of schizophrenics with positive symptoms.

Another foundation for the genetic theory is the biochemical changes in the body. The use of hallucinogens such as mescaline and LSD produce in human beings perceptions similar to Schizophrenia, and bulbocapnine can produce a catatonic like state in animals. Also 3, 4-dimethophenylathylamine, a substance similar to mescaline, has been found in the urine of many schizophrenic patients. Abnormal indoles have also been found in schizophrenics' urine, but both of these substances could have dietary origins. Abnormalities of carbohydrate metabolism are believed to be the result of secondary factors too. R. G. Heath has isolated a specific protein factor named taraxein from the serum of his patients. Taraxein is related to the alpha-globulin transporter of copper in blood plasma and is inconclusively reported to have caused psychotic symptoms in volunteers.

However, as is the case with the investigations of genetic factors in schizophrenia, the research on neurological factors in schizophrenia is hampered both by the current limits of medical science and by the heterogeneous and variable character of schizophrenic symptoms which makes it more difficult for researchers to draw clear lines between structural abnormalities and behaviors (Holzman, 1996; Wahlberg, et al., 1997).

Biological Risks

A variety of environmental and biological risk factors have been associated with a greater incidence of schizophrenia. Supporting the hypothesis of genetic links in schizophrenia, the risk of developing the disorder is higher among persons who have relatives with the disorder, particularly one or more first-degree relatives (APA, 1997, p. 6). The prevalence of schizophrenia in first-degree family members is estimated at between 3.5% and 8% (low compared to many other hereditary disorders, but high compared to general population risk) (Holzman, 1996, p. 118).

On balance, there is no doubt that schizophrenia has a large genetic component—family, twin and adoptive studies demonstrates that schizophrenia runs in the biological families of patients even in cases when they are reared apart from those families (Holzman, 1996; Vallada & Kunugi, 1996; Kendler, et al., 1996; Wahlberg, et al., 1997).

There are a number of investigators who consider heredity as an important factor in the origin of Schizophrenia. Among these investigators are H. Luxenburger in Germany, E. Essen-Moller in Sweden, F. J. Kalleman and Jon L. Karlsson in the United States, and Eliot Slater in Great Britain. This notion is very unacceptable to the public and also to those who are trying to cure and rehabilitate schizophrenics, as it is quite fatalistic and the tendency of people who believe in the inheritance factor is to label schizophrenics as lost.

There are a number of different theories about the exact way in which the tendency to inheritance of Schizophrenia is passed on. Jon L. Karlsson did a convincing study in Iceland, an excellent controlled study group because of the stability of the population and the existence of census records that go back at least 150 years and sometimes much longer. These census records record those persons who are mentally ill.

The starting point of Karlsson's theory is the fact that if one combines the statistics for manic-depressive and schizophrenics, the incidence of these conditions occurring is remarkably constant. He justifies this combination by the overlapping occurrence of these two conditions in the same persons at different stages of their lives. The second supporting fact of the genetic theory is the higher incidence of schizophrenics in the same families. To control this for environmental similarities, Karlsson did a study of foster children who were schizophrenic. He traced brothers and sisters of these children who were reared away from home and discovered that the biological siblings had a predictable higher incidence of Schizophrenia than did the foster sisters and brothers reared in the same home. He has also traced mental illness through seven generations of descendents.

However, the genetic link in schizophrenia is neither as dramatic (in terms of rates of family prevalence) nor as easily identified as it is in other hereditary disorders such as Huntington's Chorea and cystic fibrosis (Holzman, 1996). In 1995, researchers located a possible abnormality on gene 6 that may be responsible for the disease. This line of thinking tends to see the disease as genetically inherited, but what, exactly, is being inherited is still unknown. For example, researchers do not know whether it is a faulty enzyme or a genetic malfunction. However, recent discoveries point to its being a genetic defect, "Researchers around the world have confirmed the general location of a gene linked to schizophrenia, the first wide-ranging scientific agreement on the existence of any gene linked to a specific mental illness."

If they're correct-and four separate labs worldwide now agree a gene affecting schizophrenia sits somewhere on chromosome six-researchers may soon be knocking on a genetic doorway that could lead to new treatment for a devastating brain illness that affects one in 100 people" (Talan, 1995: 1).

While this research has provided some evidence for a genetic schizophrenic vulnerability locus on chromosome 8p and/or chromosome 6p21-23, the genetic markers for schizophrenia have yet to be clearly identified and isolated (Kendler, et al., 1996; Vallada & Kunugi, 1996). All of this suggests that factors in addition to genetics play an important role in the etiology of schizophrenia.

Of course, there can be no treatment possible until researchers have discovered much more about the genetic defect and how to alleviate it. However, this pathway of treatment is being investigated because of the wide-ranging belief that schizophrenia is genetically based. One of the facts that makes people think this is so is that there is a higher prevalence of the disease in families that already have someone with schizophrenia in them than there is in the general population. In the general population it is one in one hundred, but it is one in 10 in families already afflicted with the disease for first—degree relatives, (Hunt, 1996). Yet, this new treatment pathway is still a long way from being a reality. The new gene discovery has caused an atmosphere of caution because "In the past, highly publicized markers for a schizophrenia gene on chromosome five were discovered but the chromosome failed to pan out. Even if scientists can isolate and clone a gene, past studies suggest that it takes more than defective genes to trigger mental decline. Research on identical twins suggests that even if both share the same genes, there is only a 50 percent chance that both will have schizophrenia" (Talan, 1995: 3).

Karlsson concluded that Schizophrenia was passed through two separate genes. He reaches this conclusion from observation that when a schizophrenic parent has children, the chances that his offspring will be schizophrenic are only 16%. However, if both parents are schizophrenic, the chances are as high as 40 to 70%. This Karlsson postulates as a gene modified dominant inheritance. He also suggests that one of the two genes responsible for Schizophrenia is also responsible for creative genius, at least in some part.

Other proponents of the genetic theory have different theories of transmission. Kallemann believes in a single recessive gene of limited manifestation. Others assume a dominant gene, and still others a multiple mode of inheritance. However, recent studies of chromosomes that confirmed the heredity nature of some types of mental deficiency did not indicate any specific chromosome alteration in schizophrenics.

Environmental Risks

While concurring that biological factors (both neurological and genetic) play a key—indeed, essential—role in the etiology of schizophrenia, contemporary researchers are also in agreement that environmental factors are in most cases at least partially implicated in the disease. Contemporary researchers tend to emphasize a vulnerability-stress model of schizophrenia, wherein genetic and/or neurological factors create an inherent vulnerability to contracting schizophrenia and stress factors in the external environment serve to "push" the person towards psychological decompensation and schizophrenia (Larsen & Opjordsmoen, 1996; APA, 1997; Wahlberg, 1997). Family, twin, and adoptive studies have for the most part reiterated the importance of the family environment in the production of schizophrenia. These study results demonstrate that highly stressful family environments and highly dysfunctional family communication patterns constitute a very strong environmental push factor in persons already at biological risk for schizophrenia (APA, 1997; Larsen & Opjordsmoen, 1996; Wahlberg, 1997). Other studies have likewise demonstrated that certain types of low-affect family communication patterns can improve outcome prognosis, while high-affect communication patterns worsen outcome prognosis (Lefley, 1997; APA, 1997).

At the same time, these studies have dispelled the myth of the "schizophrenogenic" family—the hypothesis that "a sufficiently dysfunctional rearing family could generate schizophrenic illness in almost anyone" (Wahlberg, et al., 1997, p. 360). In contrast to this hypothesis, the adoptive family studies demonstrate that persons at low or no—biological risk for schizophrenia do **not** develop the disorder even when raised in families rated as highly dysfunctional.

Identified social-environmental risk factors in schizophrenia include lower socioeconomic class, industrialized nation, urban center residence, and single (versus married) status (APA, 1997, p. 7). A number of prenatal and perinatal factors have been associated with an increased risk for developing schizophrenia. These include obstetrical complications, winter birth, Rh incompatibility, low birth weight, maternal malnutrition, and maternal exposure to the influenza virus during the second trimester of pregnancy (Wyatt, et al., 1996).

Psychological Theories

With the schizophrenias and related paranoid syndromes, psychologists argue that we move into a realm of behavioral disorder that represents in many ways the ultimate in psychological breakdown (Meise & Fleischacker, 1996). The symptoms of these disorders include the most extreme to be found in human behavior, and they include virtually all of the pathological processes identified as potentially self-destructive and dangerous to others (Litrell, Herth, & Hinte, 1996).

The psychological approach to schizophrenia views the disease as being related to the environment. There have been many environmental factors associated with contributing to the condition of schizophrenia, if not representing outright causative factors. Being raised by people who have schizophrenia and socio-economic conditions have also been linked to the disease.

Even the way families interact and communicate has been addressed as a possible factor in the evolution of the disease, "Unclear communication within families is one potential condition, although investigators are still uncertain whether this deviant communication is the cause or result of schizophrenia in a given family member. The disorganized family life often associated with poverty has also been implicated in schizophrenia; in addition, poverty may lead mothers to neglect their health, which may in turn affect the health of a fetus or newborn child" (Encarta, 1997: 1).

Sociological Theories

There are many that deny a genetic or biological causation for Schizophrenia and postulate other theories. Thomas J. Scheff postulates a sociological theory. He repudiates the basically Freudian notion that Schizophrenia is something contained within the individual, with the external world merely providing triggers. On the contrary, Scheff believes that insanity is an individual's response to the difficult situations in which he or she is placed. The model for insanity is learned in childhood. When the person deviates from normal behavior, the persons around him act as if he is crazy. Then he adopts the full mode of insanity. Seeking treatment, the individual is more firmly situated in his role. Scheff states, "These considerations suggest that the labeling process is a crucial contingency in most careers of residual deviance."

Don Jackson also points out the ways that society affects an individual's madness. He brings up the example of "wedding psychosis," the malady that affects Muslim girls when they are about to enter marriage. There are numerous other cases when the shape and the incidence of mental disease seems to spring from the culture rather than operate as a biological phenomenon.

Karl Menninger supports a more individual theory that does not fail to consider society. He sees mental illness as "personality dysfunction and living impairment." He continues,

> It sees all patients not as individuals afflicted with certain diseases but as human beings obliged to

make awkward and expensive maneuvers to maintain themselves, individuals who have become somewhat isolated from their fellows, harassed by faulty techniques of living, uncomfortable themselves, and often to others. Their reactions are intended to ¼insure survival even at the cost of suffering and disaster.

Ronald D. Laing has a popular theory that bears some relation to that of Jung. He sees the schizophrenic as searching for transcendence through self-knowledge. The mad person really sees things, but society treats him as an imbecile. Some people choose not to return to ordinary reality. Laing at present is treating people under these theories.

In conclusion, there are many theories but few facts concerning the origins of Schizophrenia. There is a basic disagreement if the disorder is basically psychological, occurring in genetic patterns, or if it is psychological resulting from environment. It is important to answer these questions, for there are many afflicted people being treated without knowledge of the cause, usually on the trial and error method.

Alternatives

Recently, there have been a number of investigations conducted into viruses as a potential causative factor of schizophrenia. This theory is controversial, but some researchers continue to investigate this area because while heredity may play a role in the development of the disease studies have shown that identical twins do not suffer from schizophrenia equally. One objection to this theory is that no research has been able to isolate a probable virus as the cause, but research has shown that drugs used to treat schizophrenia or bipolar (manic-depressive) disorder may inhibit viruses.

Those that believe schizophrenia may be caused by an unknown virus believe these types of drugs may be effective in helping inhibit the effects of the disease, and some research points in that direction. "A recent study published in Schizophrenia Research puts these casual observations on a somewhat firmer footing." Metabolic by-products of the antipsychotic drug clozapine inhibit the growth of HIV in a standard cell-culture system. Champions of the viral causation theory note that other viruses may be similarly affected by antipsychotic medicines. Conceivably, they suggest, clozapine and some other antipsychotic drugs whose mode of action is uncertain might work by suppressing an unknown virus" (Beardsley 1).

Racial Disparities

Interestingly, many studies of this theory have been conducted with members of ethnic and racial minority groups. Of late, the professional literature in the field of psychology has been focused on the question of whether or not African-Americans are at-risk for being misdiagnosed (or overly diagnosed) as schizophrenic (Coleman and Baker, 1994).

Lawson, Hepler, Holladay and Cuffel (1994) studied this issue. They used census data from 1984 and 1990 from 37 Tennessee Department of Mental Health out—and inpatient facilities to determine patterns of diagnosis for African—Americans seen by or treated in such facilities. Referring to the Diagnostic and Statistical Manual of Mental Disorders—III—Revised (DSM-III—R) criteria for diagnosis, they found that the main diagnostic categories of African-Americans were schizophrenia, alcohol and drug abuse disorders, and affective disorders. They also found that in both 1990 and 1984, the proportion of African-Americans committed to state mental health institutions (31 and 30 percent, respectively) was considerably larger than for the general population. They concluded that a tendency to overdiagnose schizophrenia among African-Americans was evident.

Worthington (1992) examined factors influencing the diagnosis and treatment of African-American patients in the mental health system. She conducted a literature review of 12 articles published since 1965 on the topic of racial and ethnic factors as they pertain to misdiagnosis and/or tendencies to focus on specific diagnoses when assessing African-Americans. Specific findings revealed an association between race and hospital diagnosis, higher rates of depression diagnosis in whites and schizophrenia diagnosis (as well as manic depression) in African—Americans. Part of the problem, in her view, is that many of the tests used to identify possible schizophrenia—including the Minnesota Multiphasic Personality Inventory (MMPI) are skewed toward and normed against Anglo-Americans and are not necessarily sensitive to African-Americans and other minorities. Other tests, such as the Allen Cognitive Levels Assessment (ACL) and the Functional Needs Assessment (FNA), do not appear to contain built-in normative biases and are more accurate in identifying schizophrenia and schizoaffective disorder.

Flaskerud and Hu (1988) conducted an extensive study, employing a sample of 24,600 adult white, African-American, Latino and Asian clients of a county mental health system. They found that African-American and Asian clients had a greater proportion of psychotic diagnoses than did whites and Latinos a lesser proportion than whites. Whites and Asians received more diagnoses of major affective disorders than did African-Americans or Latinos, and these two populations were more likely to be diagnosed as schizophrenic than either whites or Asians.

Fabrega, Mezzich, and Ulrich (1988) reported similar results. These researchers examined differences in psychopathology among 5,297 white and 1,376 African-American patients admitted to a large urban psychiatric facility. Results indicated that there was a significant variation in psychopathology associated with ethnicity, despite controlling for gender, age and education. Variation was most pronounced for unipolar depression disorders, but also included schizophrenia, paranoid/other psychoses, anxiety disorders, and dementia. Coleman and Baker (1994) reported that a pilot study with eight African-American male veterans age 51 to 77 years who were patients at a VA mental hospital demonstrated support for the view that misdiagnosis of schizophrenia is of concern in this population. They found that after two investigators separately reviewed the subjects' medical records and conducted psychiatric interviews with the subjects, seven had their diagnoses changed from schizophrenia to an affective disorder.

Concerns regarding this tendency were explored at the 2nd annual Black Task Force Conference held in San Francisco in October of 1984—an indication of how long members of the mental health profession have been concerned with this issue. Fullilove (1986) reported that it was suggested that African-Americans are overdiagnosed as schizophrenic and underdiagnosed with regard to affective disorders because of a fundamental lack of understanding and knowledge of the special pressures impacting upon the African-American family, individual and community.

Further, the situation is also an artifact of the use of test and assessment instruments normed to the white community and not sensitive to the cultural nuances of the African-American community. Ruiz (1985) also explored this particular explanation of the causes of this problem. He found that minority patients treated in American mental health facilities might differ in symptomatology of such illnesses as affective disorders and schizophrenia. Language and cultural differences that impede understanding of minority populations are of some significance in fostering possible misdiagnosis of schizophrenia and other conditions. He argued that it is now necessary to rethink the conceptual model of defining and classifying mental health and mental illness and to take into consideration ethnic differences, cultural characteristics, and social factors.

Jones and Gray (1986) also sought explanations for over—or misdiagnosis of schizophrenia among African-Americans and other ethnic and racial minorities. They found several contributing factors, including the over-reliance on the classic thought disorder symptoms as pathogenic for schizophrenia. With affective disorders, the lack of clearly defined boundaries between normal and abnormal mood and a failure to realize that patients with affective illness can manifest cognitive symptoms. Misdiagnosis of schizophrenia among African-Americans also results from such factors as differences in language and mannerisms, difficulties in relating between African-American patients and white therapists, and the myth that African-Americans rarely suffer from affective disorders. These authors suggested that clinicians and researchers must pay more attention to the effects of cultural differences on diagnosis and baseline behaviors and symptomatology specific to African-Americans (and other minorities as well) must be established.

Other early research in this area also offers insight into the issue. Chu and Sallach (1900) studied the symptomatology of white and black schizophrenics and found significant differences between the two groups. Findings indicated that African—Americans exhibited more frequent symptoms of angry outbursts, poor communication, disorientation, asocial behavior, and auditory and visual hallucinations tan whites. Whites showed more frequent symptoms of unsystematized delusions.

Taken as a whole, these studies—which represent a far more substantial body of research than can be described in a report of this brevity—strongly support the belief that schizophrenia is both misdiagnosed and overdiagnosed among African-Americans.

Characteristics of Schizophrenia

Schizophrenia is not a clearly definable unified disorder. There is no "typical" schizophrenic. The psychopathology is heterogenous and multidimensional (Lindenmayer, et al., 1995). As the American Psychological Association's practice guidelines for schizophrenia caution, "the disorder is noted for great heterogeneity across individuals and variability within individuals over time" (APA, 1997, p. 5). Schizophrenia is most often conceptualized as a syndrome—a "proposed cluster of signs and symptoms whose antecedents are unknown"—involving multiple psychological processes (e.g., perceptions, ideation, feelings, behavior, motivation, attention, cognition, concentration, etc.) (Larsen and Opjordsmoen, 1996, p. 371). The psychological and behavioral characteristics of schizophrenia (e.g., hallucinations, delusions, loose associations, flatness, catatonia, disorganization, paranoia, impaired intention, etc.) are associated with a wide variety of impairments in multiple domains of functioning (e.g., self-care, working, interpersonal relationships, learning, etc.). They are also associated with an increased incidence of general medical illness (e.g., substance abuse, smoking-related disorders such as emphysema, antipsychotic-induced movement disorders, problems related to poor self-care), associated psychological disorders (e.g., depression, dissociative disorders, obsessive-compulsive disorder), and mortality, particularly from suicide (APA, 1997, Holzman, 1996; Larsen and Opjordsmoen, 1996).

Cognitive Deficit Model

Although the specific clinical features of schizophrenia vary widely across individuals and within individuals over time, and are frequently quite diverse, as noted above, clinical descriptions and analysis of schizophrenia have often focused on the structure of cognition and affect in schizophrenia. As summarized by Carter and Flesher (1995):

> A recurrent theme is the description of failure to engage in *active effortful processing*. Schizophrenic patients seem to lack the energy or will to actively organize cognition. Additionally, there is a failure to chunk, to cognitively organize information for later retrieval... Schizophrenic patients, as such, tend to be passive processors of information.... (Carter and Flesher, 1995, p. 211).

Support for this "cognitive deficit" model of schizophrenia comes from empirical studies demonstrating that adults with schizophrenia show impaired performance on tests of general intellectual functioning (Russell, et al., 1997). While it is now fairly well established that schizophrenics demonstrate impaired and/or substandard performance on a variety of measures of intellectual functioning, the long-held view that schizophrenia is a degenerative disease leading to progressive decline in intellectual functioning over the life span has been largely debunked (Russell, et al., 1997; Larsen and Opjordsmoen, 1996; Carter and Flesher,

1995; Smith, et al., 1995). Although schizophrenia is typically a chronic condition, and even though full recovery is extremely uncommon, recent studies have demonstrated that schizophrenia is not, *per se*, a progressive, degenerative disorder, at least in terms of intellectual functioning (Larsen and Opjordsmoen, 1996). As Russell, et al. (1997) found in their study, the intellectual deficits observed in schizophrenics are lifelong, both pre-dating the onset of schizophrenia and failing to show any evidence of worsening over time (p. 635).

Personality Characteristics

In addition to its particular associations with intellectual functioning and certain intellectual deficits, schizophrenia has long been associated with certain personality characteristics, although the exact nature of these associations continue to generate controversy (Smith, et al., 1995; Carter and Flesher, 1995; Larsen and Opjordsmoen, 1996). Some of the traits and behaviors commonly considered characteristic of schizophrenia include social detachment and isolation, idiosyncratic behavior, suspiciousness, an inability to form close relationships, and cognitive and perceptual distortions (Smith, et al, 1995, p. 104).

Symptoms

There are many different symptoms of schizophrenia, but not all of them are found in all patients who suffer from the disease. Usually, the characteristics of the individual that are most affected because of the disease are their thoughts, perceptions, feelings, movements and relationships with others. All of these are generally negatively affected to some degree or another.

Hallucinations—particularly hearing one's thoughts spoken aloud or hearing imaginary voices giving commands or making comments—are the principal perceptual problems. Emotional reactions to a situation appear to observers to be either flat or inappropriate. Disturbances in movement may appear as catatonia, or as apparently purposeless repetitive ones. Relationships with others are usually disturbed, often because the schizophrenic person tends to be withdrawn" (Encarta, 1997: 1).

Historically, the spectrum of symptoms characterizing have been conceptualized as falling into two broad categories: 1) positive (active, florid psychosis) and 2) negative (or deficit) symptoms (APA, 1997; Lindenmayer, et al., 1995; Larsen and Opjordsmoen, 1996). Major "positive" symptoms include delusions and hallucinations, while the major negative symptoms include poverty of speech, flatness of affect, decreased spontaneous movement, anhedonia, and decreased initiation of goal-directed behavior (APA, 1997, p. 5). This positive/negative approach to symptom classification, while useful, has been proven to have a number of limitations. As Lindenmayer (1995) and associates note: "Most schizophrenics present a mixed syndrome; the criteria for what constitutes a positive and negative syndrome are variable; distinguishing primary from secondary negative symptoms can be difficult..." (p. 23).

Coleman (1989) and Zane, Enemoto and Chun (1992) characterize that group of disorders known as the schizophrenias as a group of psychotic disorders characterized by gross distortions of reality, withdrawal from social interaction, and disorganization and fragmentation of perception, thought, and emotion. Schizophrenic disorders occur in all societies, and in the United States it is estimated that about 1 percent of the population suffers from this disorder—an indication that it is far less widespread than either bipolar disorder or depression. The schizophrenias are considered the most serious of all disorders, as well as among the most baffling. These are, ultimately, two different types of disorders; the form may or may not, dependent upon severity, be a psychotic disorder, while the latter always is. There are several types of schizophrenia identified by the APA. The first is undifferentiated type, in which indications of perplexity, confusion, emotional turmoil, delusions of reference, excitement, and dreamlike autism as well as depression and fear. In the paranoid type, symptoms are dominated by absurd, illogical, and changeable delusions, frequently accompanied by vivid hallucinations with a resulting impairment of critical judgment and erratic, unpredictable, and even dangerous behavior. The catatonic type is characterized by alternating periods of extreme withdrawal and extreme excitement. The disorganized or hebephrenic type tends to occur at an earlier age than other schizophrenias and represents a more severe disintegration of personality. The residual type of schizophrenia encompasses mild, schizophrenic symptoms shown by individuals in remission following a schizophrenic episode (Coleman, 1969; Cohen, Allen, Pollin, & Hrebec, 1972).

In the fourth edition of its Diagnostic and Statistical Manual of Mental Disorders (DSM-IV), the American Psychiatric Association added a third category, disorganized, to the previously established positive and negative categories. The disorganized symptoms include disorganized speech, disorganized behavior, and poor attention (APA, 1997, p. 5).

The three phases of schizophrenia

In assessing and treating schizophrenia, clinicians commonly divide the course of schizophrenia into three main phases: 1) acute; 2) stabilization; and 3) stable (APA, 1997, p. 6). The acute phase is one in which the patient exhibits severe psychotic symptoms, particularly those symptoms within the "positive" and "disorganized" categories. During the prodromal period leading to the active acute phase, there is often an acceleration of the negative symptoms. For example, during this prodromal phase, there may be evidence of social withdrawal, loss of interest in school or work, deterioration in self-care habits like hygiene and grooming, and outbursts of anger or bizarre behavior. During the "stabilization" phase, the acute positive and disorganized symptoms decrease in severity, while the "negative" symptoms may manifest in considerable variability. As its name implies, during the "stable phase," the symptoms are relatively stable and mild, when present at all (some patients are asymptomatic during the stable phase). Some patients may manifest other non-schizophrenic psychiatric symptoms during the stable phase (e.g., anxiety, depression, and insomnia). It should be noted that these classifications are made as an aid to assessment and treatment planning for the clinician. In the patient, these phases are often seen to merge into one another without clear boundaries.

Subtypes

In addition to classifying symptoms into types and levels of severity, clinicians follow DSM-IV criteria in grouping the schizophrenic patient into one of four major subtypes, generally defined by the predominant symptoms at the time of the most recent evaluation (hence, the subtypes can change over time). The *paranoid* subtype features a preoccupation with delusions or hallucinations; the *disorganized type* features disorganized speech and behavior, along with flat and/or inappropriate affect; and the *catatonic type* features extreme withdrawal and characteristic motor symptoms. A fourth subtype, *undifferentiated type*, is a nonspecific category used when no other subtype feature predominates (APA, 1997, p. 5). Though it is by no means clear that schizophrenia is a unitary process, psychologists tend to argue that these disorders are characterized primarily by disorganization of thought processes, a lack of coherence between thought and emotion, and an inward orientation away from reality (Meise & Fleischacker, 1996).

Comorbidity

The literature strongly suggests that while depression may play a role in the symptomatic presentation of undifferentiated schizophrenia, it is not the same disorder and is in fact significantly different from schizophrenia. Cognitive impairment in schizophrenia is known to impede psychosocial performance and eventual reintegration into society; additionally, schizophrenics tend to experience worsening of their symptoms under conditions of stress, responding negatively to common environmental and social stressors virtually impossible to avoid in mainstream society (Tollefson, 1996).

Alternative Classification

Conflicting definitions have led Lindenmayer (1995) and others to develop alternative symptom classification schemes. For example, Lindenmayer (1995) has developed a 5-factor model which includes the categories of: 1) negative component (e.g., emotional withdrawal, lack of spontaneity, poor rapport, blunted affect, social avoidance); 2) excitement component (e.g., poor impulse control, hostility, tension); 3) cognitive component (e.g., conceptual disorganization, disorientation, poor attention); 4) positive component (e.g., delusions, unusual thought content, grandiosity, suspiciousness, hallucinations); and 5) depression component (e.g., anxiety, guilt feelings, depression, somatic concerns) (p. 25).

Course of Illness

Schizophrenia has its onset before a person reaches mid-life. The first episode occurs in youth normally, but some people may have one episode and then resume a normal life. Others may have three or four episodes and then return to normal. Still, many others are plagued with the following types of symptoms for the rest of their lives, "'Thought disorders may be observed as a failure to make logical connections or by the development of delusions. The lifetime prevalence of schizophrenia varies in different populations but the results of most studies suggests that a weighted average lifetime prevalence rate for the general population is on the order of 1% (APA, 1997; Larsen & Opjordsmoen, 1996). Epidemiological studies indicate that schizophrenia is fairly evenly distributed throughout the world, although industrialized countries manifest slightly higher prevalence rates than less developed countries (Satorius, et al., 1996). In the U.S., the most recently conducted Epidemiological Catchment Area Study found that the lifetime prevalence rates varied from 0.6% to 1.9% across four U.S. sites (Los Angeles, St. Louis, Baltimore, and New Haven, Connecticut) (APA, 1997, p. 6).

Schizophrenia is for the most part a disorder of adulthood. In most cases, the onset of schizophrenia occurs in late adolescence or early adulthood, with the peak age of onset for men in the early 20s and for women in the late 20s and early 30s (APA, 1997, p. 6; Gur, et al., 1996). Childhood-onset (i.e., onset before age 12) schizophrenia is extremely rare, having about one-fiftieth the treated prevalence of adult-onset schizophrenia (Alaghband-Rad, et al., 1997).

Furthermore, childhood-onset schizophrenia, when it does occur, can be distinguished from adult-onset schizophrenia in a number of ways. Notable is that childhood onset schizophrenia tends to be of a more homogeneous character (less variability in symptoms and presentation than seen in adults). Another noteworthy finding from the research literature is the evidence for a stronger neurobiological basis for early-onset schizophrenia (e.g., greater evidence of cerebral damage, greater intensity of symptoms) (Alaghband-Rad, et al., 1997).

Over the course of a lifetime, schizophrenia affects men and women with equal frequency, although the age of onset for males (early 20s) is typically earlier than for females (late 20s) (APA, 1997; Gur, et al., 1996). Although there are no major gender differences in the lifetime prevalence of schizophrenia, there are significant gender differences in the symptom dimensions of schizophrenia across the life span. Based on their study of 272 schizophrenic patients (divided into four age groups ranging from under 35 years to over 85 years), Gur, et al (1996) found a greater severity of negative symptoms in men (versus schizophrenic women) for all but the 8th decade, when the trend reversed and women were found to have greater severity of negative symptoms (p. 9). These researchers found no gender differences in the severity of positive symptoms across the life span, with the exception previously noted in other studies of the earlier onset of symptoms in males.

Although a small minority of schizophrenics remain symptom-free (or relatively so) following an initial acute episode, for most individuals, schizophrenia constitutes a chronic disorder. The illness runs a variable course, with the majority of persons experiencing exacerbations and remissions, and a smaller number exhibiting chronic, unremitting severe psychosis (Holzman, 1996; APA, 1997; Wyatt, et al., 1996; Carter and Flesher, 1995). Longitudinal studies indicate that both specific and nonspecific symptoms worsen with age, although most patients show a gradual lessening of positive symptoms (e.g., hallucinations, delusions) with aging along with a worsening of negative symptoms (e.g., withdrawal, blunting of affect, etc.) (Gur, et al., 1996).

Prognosis

Schizophrenia is one of the more difficult of all disorders which can confront the social worker or psychiatrist. Garfield and Bergin (1990) have noted that schizophrenics often require either short or long-term institutionalization and care, particularly when they are in controllable states. Until relatively recent times, the prognosis for schizophrenia was generally unfavorable; most patients diagnosed with this disorder were likely to be maintained almost permanently in mental institutions, where the rate of discharge was about 30 percent.

The current outlook has been significantly improved with the introduction of the phenothiazines (major tranquillizing drugs) in the 1950s. Chemotherapy, together with other modern treatment methods, permits the majority of cases to be treated in outpatient clinics (Aberg-Wistedt, Cressell, Lidberg, & Liljenberg, 1995).

Researchers have identified a number of prognostic variables that are useful in predicting long-term outcome in individual cases. In general, better outcomes (i.e., lower frequency of acute episodes, lower intensity of symptoms) are associated with female gender, family history of affective disorder, no family history of schizophrenia, higher IQ, married marital status, low-affect communication patterns in the living environment, good premorbid functioning, fewer prior episodes, paranoid subtype, a greater predominance of positive versus negative symptoms, living in a developing versus developed country, early treatment, and minimal comorbidity (APA, 1997; Gur, et al., 1996; Satorius, et al., 1996; Lefley, 1997).

Treatment

Even though increasingly effective medication treatments for schizophrenia have been developed, psychiatric researchers have not yet arrived at a medication protocol which can provide reliable and safe relief of symptoms to all schizophrenics (APA, 1997; Holzman, 1996; Wyatt, Apud, and Potkin, 1996). Coleman (1986) points out that the affective disorders are mood disorders in which extreme and inappropriate levels of mood—manifested as extreme elation or as deep depression—dominate the clinical picture. By contrast, schizophrenic and paranoid disorders are predominantly disturbances of thought, though they often present some distortion of affect as well. A disorder of the thought processes is not usually a notable feature in affective disorders, however, except perhaps where the disorder reaches extreme intensity. Even here the disturbed thinking often seems in some sense "appropriate" to the extremes of motion that the person is experiencing.

Treatment of these disorders is complicated by the very nature of the illness itself; Meise and Fleischacker (1996) have noted that this treatment generally involves the integration of biological, psychosocial, and environmental factors within a comprehensive treatment plan. While the majority of all schizophrenics typically participate in some type of ongoing (even life-long) psychotherapy, some success in using non-pharmaceutical treatments (alone or in combination with drug therapy) and interventions has been observed.

Currently, all available treatment for schizophrenia is inherently palliative, versus curative or preventive (APA, 1997; Wyatt, et al., 1996; Larsen & Opjordsmoen, 1996; Mattes, 1997). The scope and intensity of the treatment protocol is geared around the specific phase (acute, stabilization, stable) of the disease within the individual. Regardless of the phase of illness, all treatment plans for schizophrenia encompass the following: 1) establishing and maintaining a therapeutic alliance (essential both to accurate assessment of psychiatric status and to the facilitation of patient treatment compliance); 2) on-going psychiatric assessment and monitoring of the patient's psychiatric status (owing to the episodic, phase-driven nature of the disorder); 3) pharmacologic treatment (used in the treatment of acute episodes, the prevention of future episodes, and the improvement of symptoms between episodes); 4) medical/physical status monitoring and treatment (related both the co-morbid medical conditions and drug side-effect problems) and 5) psycho-social interventions (including family interventions, patient education, vocational counseling, social skills training, and cognitive therapy) (APA, 1997).

There is no known cure for schizophrenia. However, there are three treatment modalities that have been used to help the schizophrenic lead some type of normal lifestyle. We can categorize these modalities into three groups: biological, psychological and chemical.

Psychological Treatments

There are some people who feel that treatment medications are actually more part of the problem than they are part of the cure. These people argue that the drugs are no better help than when people who had schizophrenia were locked up in mental wards or prison cells. They feel this way because the drugs cannot cure the disease, they can only alleviate some of its symptoms, "The drugs in question are pharmacological straight-jackets. They are not curative. In effect they resemble the mechanical restraints-locks, bars, chains-that were in use up to the middle of the nineteenth century" (Whittam Smith, 1997: 1).

Some efforts are developing behavior modification interventions which incorporate self-instructional training have been undertaken. Nevertheless, these researchers have suggested that there is little empirical evidence supporting any particular efficacy for the cognitive-behavioral interventions in the treatment of schizophrenia. Affective disorders such as bipolar affective disorder and depression are far more amenable to amelioration via cognitive behavioral therapy than are any of the schizophrenias. Both of these disorders as well as schizophrenia appear to be amenable to pharmaceutical therapies.

Traditionally, psychotherapy is bypassed in an effort to save costs, since pharmacological treatment is much less expensive. In light of this information, the future approach should be for a combination of the two treatments, and for the Department of

Health to insure that health budgets allow for the additional costs of psychotherapy for schizophrenic patients. There is a solution that, while it cannot possibly resolve the age-old mind/body dichotomy, can facilitate progress in handling schizophrenia. The method is to combine medication with therapy. Neither approach has yet been able to provide a cure, but both can alleviate the distressing symptoms of schizophrenia in their different ways. Why not use them together? In fact dual treatment has often been advocated, but rarely put into practice because the cost of psychotherapy is significantly higher than the costs of drugs. It is the sheer quantity of psychotherapeutic work that cannot often be afforded under present health budgets. Typically a psychotherapist may have to work with a single sufferer for four sessions a week over a period of two years and sometimes longer. (Whittam Smith, 1997: 2).

Chemical Treatments

The "first line" pharmacologic treatment for schizophrenia (in both the acute and stabilization phases) involves the use of anti-psychotic medications, which include so-called conventional antipsychotics (also called "neuroleptics) such as fluphenazine, mesoridazine, haloperidol, and thioridazine; newer "atypical antipsychotics" such as clozapine and resperidone; and other new but as yet unmarketed (not yet approved by the FDA) anti-psychotics such as olanzapine, sertindole, and quetiapine. While there are individual differences in response to anti-psychotic medications, and although these medications differ in both their half-lives (the length of time a drug is active in the body) and their propensity to cause side-effects, in general studies have demonstrated that anti-psychotic medications are quite effective in eliminating and/or significantly reducing the severity of the symptoms of schizophrenia (APA, 1997; Mattes, 1997).

For example, the APA (1997) notes that 60% of schizophrenic patients treated with anti-psychotic medications for 6 weeks improve to the extent that they achieve a complete remission or experience only mild symptoms, while another 32% experience significant partial relief, and just 8% so no improvement or worsening of symptoms (p. 10).

Although anti-psychotic medications are quite effective at alleviating the symptoms of schizophrenia, they all produce a broad range of side-effects which can in many cases create significant medical problems (e.g., anemia, blood disorders, liver problems, kidney problems, neurological problems) and/or cause the patient significant personal and social impairment. Often most troubling from the patient's perspective are the "extrapyramidal side effects" which include parkinsonism, dystonia, and akathisia. These types of side-effects produce a broad range of movement-disorders, including involuntary muscle movements and muscle freezing (often occurring in the facial region, making it more obvious to observers), tremors, and compulsions related to a sense of physical restlessness (APA, 1997; Mattes, 1997).

To treat both the side-effects of anti-psychotic medications and to alleviate comorbid symptoms not addressed by these drugs, clinicians typically utilize a wide range of "adjunct" medications in the treatment of schizophrenia. These include beta-blockers, calcium channel blockers (to reduce movement disorder problems), tranquilizers (to alleviate anxiety and reduce movement disorder problems), anti-depressants (primarily tricyclic antidepressants to alleviate depression), and lithium and the anticonvulsants such as valproate and carbamazapine (to address manic symptoms) (APA, 1997; Wyatt, et al., 1996; Mattes, 1997).

Medication has become the most common method of treating schizophrenia because the prevailing theories over its cause have shifted in the past three decades from environmental causes to brain chemistry. Instead of believing that the diseases is caused by environmental factors, most experts now feel that brain chemistry imbalances and genetics play the greatest role in the development of the disease, "Nowadays giving drugs to schizophrenic patients is often the sole method used to control the illness. The prevailing view is that schizophrenia is organic in nature, and diseases of the brain are probably genetic in origin. The patient is disabled and requires a sheltered environment plus medication. This contrasts with the conventional wisdom of thirty years ago when stressful events in early childhood were believed to he a major factor. In its crudest formulation, it was said that families causes schizophrenia" (Whittam Smith, 1997: 1).

These and other theories continue to be investigated as more technology becomes available that allows us to more accurately explore the human brain and its functioning. The types of drugs that are presently used to help ameliorate the effects of schizophrenia have a tranquilizing effect on the patient. They are sedative in nature and often will cause a decrease in episodes and a lessening of anxiety. In this context, Coleman (1986) notes that the phenothiazines (major tranquilizing drugs) have been useful in treating the schizophrenia and in eliminating the need, in many cases, for long-term institutionalization. However, the rate of readmissions among diagnosed schizophrenics who are on prophylactic pharmaceutical regimens is about 45 percent within the first year after release. Overall, about one-third of schizophrenic patients recovers while another third show partial recovery while another third remain largely or totally disabled.

Combination Treatments

While first—and second-line medications constitute a primary treatment modality in all schizophrenia, a wide variety of psychosocial treatment interventions are also commonly used. These interventions, which include family therapy, patient education, social skills training, individual therapy, and vocational counseling among others, aim broadly at helping the schizophrenic patient to adjust to daily living and re-integrate to society following an acute episode and/or during periods of stability.

Littrell, Herth and Hinte (1996) examined the effects of psychosocial treatment and clopazine therapy with a population of 44 patients with refractory schizophrenia and a history of suicide attempts. They found that patients treated with both types of intervention—chemical and non-chemical—tended to progress more rapidly, exhibit a higher level of hope for an eventual reintegration into the social and communal mainstream, and demonstrate a reduction in symptoms as well as decreased suicidality. Patients who received only one of the interventions were less likely to exhibit these attitudinal and behavioral changes.

Studies of treatment with and without chemotherapy also have been identified in the literature. Mosak (1995) offered an analysis of two case studies to demonstrate that therapists do not necessarily need to utilize drugs in treating schizophrenics. His view is that psychologists and psychiatrists tend to become overly dependent upon pharmaceutical treatment when working with this population. Nevertheless, Schwartzberg, Wheelis, and Zarate (1996) have countered by presenting results of several cases in which initial treatment of schizophrenia incorporated the use of clozapine and in which withdrawal of the drug was followed by a period of decomposition and a return to symptomology.

Future Research

Because of the lack of a cure and because of the controversy that surrounds most of the treatment options for schizophrenia, there are new paths of study and research being explored all the time. Once such explorer is a young scientist who won a half-million dollar grant to continue the studies she researched in college about the cause of this disease. Her motivation to study psychology and this disease stem from the fact that her sister is a diagnosed schizophrenic, and she suffered in pain as she watched her beloved sister struggle with this disease. She realized she and her brother had different blood types than her afflicted sister, who was incompatible with their mother's blood type (as they were not).

Thus, Meggin Hollister decided to test her theories while attending the University of Southern California, "Meggin decided to test a hunch that incompatibility between Rh-negative mothers and their Rh-positive fetuses might be a factor in causing schizophrenia. Her hypothesis was that the mother produces antibodies to attack the foreign blood antigens, which, when coupled with a genetic predisposition, may affect the baby's brain development. Since 1968, drugs have been routinely used to stop production of such antibodies" (Rogers & McNeil, 1996: 2).

Limitations of Research

Research on schizophrenia has occurred for more than a century, and intensive efforts have been undertaken for the past three decades. However, most of this research has come to nothing. Yet, one of the biggest obstacles may be that researchers are very often not in contact with the actual sufferers of schizophrenia (as Meggin Hollister was). As such, all too often the experiences and words of the schizophrenic have been ignored as having any value that could add to the discovery process. "Researchers in this field, cut off as they are from actual patients, adamantly refuse to attribute any significance to what sufferers from schizophrenia might say about themselves. Their hallucinations, their delusions, their strange talk, their inexplicable silences, their thought disorders are all dismissed as the meaningless results of convulsive electric brain storms. Attempts to make sense of schizophrenic discourse are seen as a waste of time," (Whittam Smith, 1997: 2).

Rehabilitation

Rehabilitation for schizophrenics is now a multi-faceted intervention approach that incorporates chemotherapy, vocational training, and behavior modification techniques (Aberg-Wistedt, et al, 1995). For—these reasons, reintegrations of the schizophrenic into society is at best a difficult task and, at worst an often-impossible one. With more than one million actively schizophrenic patients currently known to live in the United States, and only about 600,000 being treated at any given time in medical or psychological care settings, the question of social reintegration is one of some concern (Schaub, Aridres, Brenner, & Donzel, 1997).

Given that vocational disabilities often are linked to this disorder, a return to productive, functional integration into society (including work and family life) is often tenuous at best. Hodel and Bettina (1997) have identified the conditions associated with favorable outcomes in the treatment of schizophrenia. These include:

1. Reactive rather than process schizophrenia, in which the time from onset of symptoms is 6 or fewer months;
2. Clear-cut precipitating stressors;
3. Good social, work, and heterosexual adjustment prior to schizophrenic episode;
4. Minimal incidence of this and other pathologies in family history;

5. Involvement of depression or other schizophrenic pattern;
6. Good or favorable life situation to return to and adequate aftercare in the community.

Thus, both pre—and post-episode factors are known to impinge directly upon the course of the disorder and the reintegration of the schizophrenic. In general, the opposite of the foregoing conditions (including poor premorbid adjustment, slow onset, a familial history of the disorder, and a lack of an adequate community or family support system) are counter-indicative of a positive course of treatment or return pattern (Hodel & Bettina, 1997).

Similarly, Meise and Fleischacker (1996) have also argued that a combined treatment approach, employing both neuroleptic and antipsychotic drugs, is often beneficial in facilitating a return to work, community and family. Critical variables known to impact upon treatment efficacy include severity and duration of the schizophrenic episode(s), and the nature and extent of vocational disability.

At issue in a return to mainstream life is the question of vocational rehabilitation; for the schizophrenic whose disorder is "under control" because of pharmaceutical treatment, it is vitally important to include a vocational rehabilitation component in treatment protocols. In this context, Lehman (1995) states that most vocational rehabilitation programs designed for use with this population have historically had a positive influence on work-related activities, but most have failed to show substantial and enduring impacts on independent, competitive employment.

This is a critical concern, given that we now live in an era of deinstitutionalization for schizophrenic patients in which many such individuals have been provided with minimal institutional services and then released back into community life. Recent advances in supported employment have suggested that vocational rehabilitation offers greater promise than transitional and sheltered employment approaches. Lehman (1995) suggests that vocational rehabilitation may exert a positive influence on such clinical outcomes as medication compliance, symptom reduction, and relapse. Aberg-Wistedt, et al. (1995) assessed two-year outcomes of 40 patients with schizophrenic disorders who were randomly assigned to either a team-based, intensive care management program or to standard psychiatric services.

The case management model featured increased staff contact time with patients, rehabilitation plans based on patients' expressed needs, and patients' attendance at team meetings where their rehabilitation plan was discussed. Patients in the case management group had significantly fewer emergency visits compared with the two-year period before the study. Their family members reported a significantly reduced burden of care associated with ongoing relationships with psychiatric services over the two-year study period. The size of patients' social networks increased for the case management group and decreased for the control group (Aberg—Wistedt, et al, 1995). These researchers concluded that for a successful return to community life and meaningful work, schizophrenics require a multimodal intervention and treatment approach.

These authors believe that a combination of chemotherapy and cognitive therapy must be understood as offering the greatest degree of hope for a full return to functional participation within the social mainstream. Hodel and Brenner (1997) also support the integration of cognitive and behavioral therapies with some type of pharmaceutical regimen in the treatment of schizophrenics. For a successful return, it is also important to ensure that the schizophrenic will reenter the world and make a close connection with significant others, including family, co-workers, and community-based treatment centers and therapists.

Given that cultural factors often influence the type, symptom content, and even the incidence of schizophrenic disorders, the social setting to which the schizophrenic is returned must be understood as a vital component in successful reintegration.

Conclusion

Schizophrenia is a disorder with a highly individualized presentation, and thus each schizophrenic must be understood and treated as a unique individual. Schizophrenia is the most devastating of all psychiatric illnesses. Its impact upon the relatively tiny proportion of the population affected by the disorder is virtually incalculable and its economic, social, and psychological impact on the immediate family, caregivers, and society as a whole is substantial.

While research over the past two decades has helped to illuminate the etiology of the disorder, clarified some of its clinical features, and led to the development of more effective treatment protocols, schizophrenia today largely remains an unsolved puzzle.

In conclusion, one can readily see that schizophrenia is not, as commonly thought, multiple personality disorder. Nor is it a favorite with defense lawyers as a means of getting clients off the hook for their irresponsible actions. Rather, it is a devastating, personal nightmare whose symptoms and afflictions more resemble a scenario from Dante's Inferno, than the traditional symptoms of the diseases we view in our daily lives. While there have been new pathways of research opened, and while there have been genetic links possibly established to pinpoint the cause of the disease, there is still no known cure.

Instead, we must rely on the traditional modes of treatment such as pharmaceuticals and psychotherapy. Both have been proven to be effective in helping to restore some quality of life to patients afflicted with this torturous disease. However, experts feel there needs to be a combined approach utilized in order to take advantage of creating the most effective treatment option. Despite decades of research and investigation into the causes and a potential cure for schizophrenia, medical science remains unable to provide us with a compelling account of what actually causes this mind-robbing disorder.

It appears that more than one cause may be responsible or that little explored avenues of research (like the viral causation theory) may play a role in the development of the disease. As new technologies become available and as more resources are spent investigating different theories, the future may yet hold the answer to the cause(s) and potential cure for this debilitating disease.

REFERENCES

Aberg-Wistedt, A., Cressell, T., Lidberg, Y., & Liljenberg, B. (1995). Two-year outcome of team-based intensive case management for patients with schizophrenia. **Psychiatric Services, 46(12)**, 1263-1266.

Alaghband-Rad, J.; Hamburger, S.D.; Giedd, J.N., et al. (1997). Childhood-onset schizophrenia: biological markers in relation to clinical characteristics. **American Journal Psychiatry**, 154 (1), 64-68.

Alaghband-Rad, J.; Hamburger, S.D.; Giedd, J.N., et al. (1997). Childhood-onset schizophrenia: biological markers in relation to clinical characteristics. **American Journal Psychiatry**, 154 (1), 64-68.

Alaghband-Rad, J.; Hamburger, S.D.; Giedd, J.N., et al. (1997). Childhood-onset schizophrenia: biological markers in relation to clinical characteristics. **American Journal Psychiatry**, 154 (1), 64-68.

American Psychiatric Association (APA) (1997). Practice guideline for the treatment of patients with schizophrenia. **American Journal Psychiatry**, 154 (4 Supplement), 1-54.

American Psychiatric Association (APA) (1997). Practice guideline for the treatment of patients with schizophrenia. **American Journal Psychiatry**, 154 (4 Supplement), 1-54.

American Psychiatric Association (APA) (1997). Practice guideline for the treatment of patients with schizophrenia. **American Journal Psychiatry**, 154 (4 Supplement), 1-54.

American Psychiatric Association. (1986). **Diagnostic and Statistical Manual of Mental Disorders.** Washington, D.C.: APA.

Aritei, S. (1955). **Interpretation of Schizophrenia.** New York: R. Brunner.

Beardsley, T. (1997). Matter Over Mind: Do Viruses Cause Severe Mental Illness? **Scientific American**, 1-2.

Beck, A.T. (1967). **Depression: Clinical, Theoretical and experimental.** New York: Harper & Row.

Carter, M. & Flesher, S. (1995). The neurosociology of schizophrenia: vulnerability and functional disability. **Psychiatry**, 58 (August), 209-224.

Carter, M. & Flesher, S. (1995). The neurosociology of schizophrenia: vulnerability and functional disability. **Psychiatry**, 58 (August), 209-224.

Carter, M. & Flesher, S. (1995). The neurosociology of schizophrenia: vulnerability and functional disability. **Psychiatry**, 58 (August), 209-224.

Chu, C., & Sallach, H. (1985). Differences in psychopathology among black and white schizophrenics. **International Journal of Social Psychiatry, 31(4),** 252—257.

Cohen, S.M., Allen, M.G., Pollini, W., & Hrtibec, Z. (1972). Relationship of schizo-affective Psychosis To Manic Depression And Schizophrenia. **Archives of General Psychiatry, 26(6),** 539-546.

Coleman, D., & Baker, F. (1994). Misdiagnosis of Schizophrenia in Older, Black veterans. **Journal of Nervous and Mental Disease, 182(9),** 527-528. Chang, E.C. (1996). Cultural Differences in Optimism, Pessimism, and Coping. **Journal of Counseling Psychology, 44(1),** 113-123.

Coleman, J.C. (1989). **Abnormal Psychology and Modern Life.** Evanston, IL: Scott, Foresman and Co.

Davison G.C., & Neale, J.M. (1986). **Abnormal Psychology.** New York: John Wiley and Sons.

Dietz, P. (1998). Perspective On Mental Illness. **Los Angeles Times. Jan. 25,** 1-3.

Fabrega, H., Mezzich, J., & Ulrich, R. (1966). Black-White Differences In Psychopathology In An Urban Psychiatric Population. **Comprehensive Psychiatry 29(3),** 265-297.

Fine, R. (1989). **A History of Psychoanalysis.** New York: Columbia University Press.

Flaskerud, J., & Eu, L. (1992). Relationship Of Ethnicity To Psychiatric Diagnosis. **Journal of Nervous and Mental Disease, 180(5),** 296-303.

Fullilove, M. (1986). Healing the Lineage. **American Journal of Social Psychiatry, 6(1),** 3-5.

Garfield, S.L. & Bergin, A.E. (1990). **Handbook of Psychotherapy and Behavior Change.** New York: John Wiley and Sons.

Gur, R.E.; Petty, R.G.; Turetsky, B.E., Gur, R.C. (1996). Schizophrenia throughout life: sex differences in severity and profile of symptoms. **Schizophrenia Research,** 21, 1-12.

Gur, R.E.; Petty, R.G.; Turetsky, B.E., Gur, R.C. (1996). Schizophrenia throughout life: sex differences in severity and profile of symptoms. **Schizophrenia Research,** 21, 1-12.

Gur, R.E.; Petty, R.G.; Turetsky, B.E., Gur, R.C. (1996). Schizophrenia throughout life: sex differences in severity and profile of symptoms. **Schizophrenia Research,** 21, 1-12.

Hanes, K.R.; Andrewes, D.G.; Pantelis, C.; & Chiu, E. (1996). Subcortical dysfunction in schizophrenia: a comparison with Parkinson's disease and Huntington's disease. **Schizophrenia Research,** 19, 121-128.

Hanes, K.R.; Andrewes, D.G.; Pantelis, C.; & Chiu, E. (1996). Subcortical dysfunction in schizophrenia: a comparison with Parkinson's disease and Huntington's disease. **Schizophrenia Research,** 19, 121-128.

Hanes, K.R.; Andrewes, D.G.; Pantelis, C.; & Chiu, E. (1996). Subcortical dysfunction in schizophrenia: a comparison with Parkinson's disease and Huntington's disease. **Schizophrenia Research**, 19, 121-128.

Hodel, B., & Brenner, H.D. (1997). A new development in integrated psychological therapy for schizophrenia patients. In H.D. Brenner, W. Boker, & R. Genner, Eds., **Towards a Comprehensive Therapy for Schizophrenia**. Gottingen, Germany: Hogrefe & Huber, 118-134.

Holzman, P.S. (1996). On the trail of the genetics and pathophysiology of schizophrenia. **Psychiatry**, 59 (May), 117-127.

Holzman, P.S. (1996). On the trail of the genetics and pathophysiology of schizophrenia. **Psychiatry**, 59 (May), 117-127.

Holzman, P.S. (1996). On the trail of the genetics and pathophysiology of schizophrenia. **Psychiatry**, 59 (May), 117-127.

Hunt, L. (1996). "The Simple Facts On Split Brain Disorder." **Independent**. Jan. 16, 1-3.

Jackson, D. D. (1964). **Myths of Madness**. Macmillian Company, New York.

Jones, B., & Gray, B. (1966). Problems in diagnosing schizophrenia and affective disorders among blacks. **Hospital and Community Psychiatry, 37(1)**, 61-65.

Jung, C. G. (1956). **Two Essays on Analytical Psychology**, Translated by R.F.C. Hull. New York: The World Publishing Company.

Karlsson, J. L. (1966). **The Biological Basis of Schizophrenia.** Springfield, Illinois: Lcharles C. Thomas.

Kendler, K.S.; MacLean, C.J.; O'Neill, A.; Burke, J., et al (1996). Evidence for a schizophrenia vulnerability locus on chromosome 8p in the Irish study of high-density schizophrenia families. **American Journal of Psychiatry**, 153 (12), 1534-1540.

Kendler, K.S.; MacLean, C.J.; O'Neill, A.; Burke, J., et al (1996). Evidence for a schizophrenia vulnerability locus on chromosome 8p in the Irish study of high-density schizophrenia families. **American Journal of Psychiatry**, 153 (12), 1534-1540.

Kendler, K.S.; MacLean, C.J.; O'Neill, A.; Burke, J., et al (1996). Evidence for a schizophrenia vulnerability locus on chromosome 8p in the Irish study of high-density schizophrenia families. **American Journal of Psychiatry**, 153 (12), 1534-1540.

Laing, R. D. & Esterton, A. (1965). **Sanity, Madness, and the Family.** New York: Basic Books.

Larsen, T.K. & Opjordsmoen, S. (1996). Early identification and treatment of schizophrenia: conceptual and ethical considerations. **Psychiatry**, 59 (Winter), 371-380.

Larsen, T.K. & Opjordsmoen, S. (1996). Early identification and treatment of schizophrenia: conceptual and ethical considerations. **Psychiatry**, 59 (Winter), 371-380.

Larsen, T.K. & Opjordsmoen, S. (1996). Early identification and treatment of schizophrenia: conceptual and ethical considerations. **Psychiatry**, 59 (Winter), 371-380.

Lawson, W., Hepler, N., Holladay, J., & Cuffel, B. (1994). Race a factor in inpatient and outpatient admissions and diagnosis. **Hospital and Community Psychiatry, 45(1),** 72-74.

Lefley, H.P. (1997). The consumer recovery vision: will it alleviate family burden? **American Journal of Orthopsychiatry,** 67 (2), 210-219.

Lefley, H.P. (1997). The consumer recovery vision: will it alleviate family burden? **American Journal of Orthopsychiatry,** 67 (2), 210-219.

Lefley, H.P. (1997). The consumer recovery vision: will it alleviate family burden? **American Journal of Orthopsychiatry,** 67 (2), 210-219.

Lehman, A.F. (1995). Vocational rehabilitation in schizophrenia. **Schizophrenia Bulletin, 21 (4),** 645-656.

Lindenmayer, J.P.: Berstein-Hyman, R.; Grochowski, S.; & Bark, N. (1995). Psychopathology of schizophrenia: initial validation of a 5-factor model. **Psychopathology,** 28, 22-31.

Lindenmayer, J.P.: Berstein-Hyman, R.; Grochowski, S.; & Bark, N. (1995). Psychopathology of schizophrenia: initial validation of a 5-factor model. **Psychopathology,** 28, 22-31.

Lindenmayer, J.P.: Berstein-Hyman, R.; Grochowski, S.; & Bark, N. (1995). Psychopathology of schizophrenia: initial validation of a 5-factor model. **Psychopathology,** 28, 22-31.

Littrell, K.H., Herth, K.A., & Hinte, L.E. (1996). The experience of hope in adults with schizophrenia. **Psychiatric Rehabilitation Journal, 19(4),** 61-65.

Mattes, J.A. (1997). Risperidone: how good is the evidence for efficacy? **Schizophrenia Bulletin,** 23 (1), 155-161.

Mattes, J.A. (1997). Risperidone: how good is the evidence for efficacy? **Schizophrenia Bulletin,** 23 (1), 155-161.

Mattes, J.A. (1997). Risperidone: how good is the evidence for efficacy? **Schizophrenia Bulletin,** 23 (1), 155-161.

Meise, U., & Fleischacker, W. 1996. Perspectives on treatment needs in schizophrenia. **British Journal of Psychiatry, 168(29),** 9-16.

Menninger, Karl. (1963). **The Vital Balance.** New York: Viking Press.

Mosak, H.H. (1995). Drugless psychotherapy with schizophrenics. Individual Psychology. **Journal of Adlerian Theory, Research, and Practice, 51 (1),** 61-66.

Rogers, P. & McNeil, I. (1996). "A Sense Of Purpose Inspired By A Sister's Schizophrenia." **People,** July 15, 1-3.

Ruiz, P. (1965). The minority patient. **Community Mental Health Journal, 21(3),** 206—216.

Russell, A.J.; Munro, J.C.; Jones, P.B., et al. (1997). Schizophrenia and the myth of intellectual decline. **American Journal Psychiatry,** 154 (5), 635-639.

Russell, A.J.; Munro, J.C.; Jones, P.B., et al. (1997). Schizophrenia and the myth of intellectual decline. **American Journal Psychiatry**, 154 (5), 635-639.

Russell, A.J.; Munro, J.C.; Jones, P.B., et al. (1997). Schizophrenia and the myth of intellectual decline. **American Journal Psychiatry**, 154 (5), 635-639.

Sartorius, N.; Gulbinat, W.; Harrison, G.; Laska, E.; & Siegel, C. (1996). Long-term follow-up of schizophrenia in 16 countries. **Social Psychiatry & Psychiatric Epidemiology**, 31, 249-258.

Sartorius, N.; Gulbinat, W.; Harrison, G.; Laska, E.; & Siegel, C. (1996). Long-term follow-up of schizophrenia in 16 countries. **Social Psychiatry & Psychiatric Epidemiology**, 31, 249-258.

Sartorius, N.; Gulbinat, W.; Harrison, G.; Laska, E.; & Siegel, C. (1996). Long-term follow-up of schizophrenia in 16 countries. **Social Psychiatry & Psychiatric Epidemiology**, 31, 249-258.

Schaub, A., Andres, K., Brenner, H.D., & Donzel, G. (1997). Developing a group format coping-oriented treatment program for schizophrenic patients. In H.D. Brenner, W. Boker, and R. Genner, Eds., **Towards a Comprehensive Therapy for Schizophrenia**. Gottingen, Germany: Hogrefe & Huber, 228-251.

Scheff, T. J. (1966). **Being Mentally Ill: A Sociological Theory.** Chicago: Aldine Publishing Company.

Schwartzberg, S., Wheelis, J., & Zarate, C.A. 1996. The danger of hopefulness: A clozapine "cure" of chronic psychosis. **Harvard Review of Psychiatry,** 4(3), 146-152.

Smith, T.E.; Shea, M.T.; Schooler, N.R.; Levin, H.; Deutsch, A.; & Grabstein, E. (1995). Studies of schizophrenia: personality traits in schizophrenia. **Psychiatry,** 58 (May), 99-113.

Smith, T.E.; Shea, M.T.; Schooler, N.R.; Levin, H.; Deutsch, A.; & Grabstein, E. (1995). Studies of schizophrenia: personality traits in schizophrenia. **Psychiatry,** 58 (May), 99-113.

Smith, T.E.; Shea, M.T.; Schooler, N.R.; Levin, H.; Deutsch, A.; & Grabstein, E. (1995). Studies of schizophrenia: personality traits in schizophrenia. **Psychiatry,** 58 (May), 99-113.

Sullivan, H. S. (1953). **Interpretation of Schizophrenia.** New York: Norton.

Talan, J. (1997). "Path To Treatment." **Newsday,** Oct. 31, 1-3.

Tien, A.Y.; Eaton, W.W.; Schlaepfer, T.E., et al. (1996). Exploratory factor analysis of MRI brain structure measures in schizophrenia. **Schizophrenia Research,** 19, 93-101.

Tien, A.Y.; Eaton, W.W.; Schlaepfer, T.E., et al. (1996). Exploratory factor analysis of MRI brain structure measures in schizophrenia. **Schizophrenia Research,** 19, 93-101.

Tien, A.Y.; Eaton, W.W.; Schlaepfer, T.E., et al. (1996). Exploratory factor analysis of MRI brain structure measures in schizophrenia. **Schizophrenia Research,** 19, 93-101.

Tollefson, G.D. (1996). Cognitive function in schizophrenic patients. **Journal of Clinical Psychiatry, 57(11), 31-39.**

Vallada, H.P. & Kunugi, H. (1996). A overview of schizophrenia genetic research presented at 1995 World Congress on Psychiatric Genetics, Cardiff. **Schizophrenia Research**, 19, 87-92.

Vallada, H.P. & Kunugi, H. (1996). A overview of schizophrenia genetic research presented at 1995 World Congress on Psychiatric Genetics, Cardiff. **Schizophrenia Research**, 19, 87-92.

Vallada, H.P. & Kunugi, H. (1996). A overview of schizophrenia genetic research presented at 1995 World Congress on Psychiatric Genetics, Cardiff. **Schizophrenia Research**, 19, 87-92.

Wahlberg, K.E.; Wynne, L.C.; Oja, H., et al. (1997). Gene-environment interaction in vulnerability to schizophrenia: findings from the Finnish adoptive family study of schizophrenia. **American Journal of Psychiatry**, 154 (3), 355-361.

Wahlberg, K.E.; Wynne, L.C.; Oja, H., et al. (1997). Gene-environment interaction in vulnerability to schizophrenia: findings from the Finnish adoptive family study of schizophrenia. **American Journal of Psychiatry**, 154 (3), 355-361.

Wahlberg, K.E.; Wynne, L.C.; Oja, H., et al. (1997). Gene-environment interaction in vulnerability to schizophrenia: findings from the Finnish adoptive family study of schizophrenia. **American Journal of Psychiatry**, 154 (3), 355-361.

Whittam Smith, A. (1997). "The Point Is Not What Causes Schizophrenia, But How To Control." **Independent**, Oct. 21, 1-3.

Worthington, C. (1992). An examination of the factors influencing diagnosis and treatment of Black patients in the mental health system. Archives of Psychiatric Nursing,6(3), 195-204.

Wyatt, R.J.; Apud, J.A.; & Potkin, S. (1996). New directions in the prevention and treatment of schizophrenia: a biological perspective. **Psychiatry**, 59 (Winter), 357-369. (1997). Schizophrenia: Public Information. **American Psychiatric Association**. Jan. 9, 1996, 1-15. "Schizophrenia." Microsoft Encarta. CD-ROM, 1.

Wyatt, R.J.; Apud, J.A.; & Potkin, S. (1996). New directions in the prevention and treatment of schizophrenia: a biological perspective. **Psychiatry**, 59 (Winter), 357-369.

Wyatt, R.J.; Apud, J.A.; & Potkin, S. (1996). New directions in the prevention and treatment of schizophrenia: a biological perspective, **Psychiatry**, 59 (Winter), 357-369.

Zane, N., Enomoto, K., & Chun, C.A. (1994). Treatment outcomes of Asian and white American clients. **Journal of Community Psychology, 22** (2), 177-191.

Zhang, D. (1995). Depression and culture: The Chinese Perspective. **Canadian Journal of Counseling, 29(3)**, 227-233.